August 25, 2017

I first met Alyssa when she was 6, a frightened little girl with flurries of seizures that stubbornly resisted treatment. A left medial temporal blush on her MRI suggested a focus for future trouble. I try to demystify epilepsy by being matter of fact in my explanations, never quite sure what people are prepared to hear, especially soon after diagnosis. But I think Alyssa was taking it all in, and years later she related her memories and impressions of those days, of course more vivid than mine. Alyssa has kept an amazing record of her experiences, a record of everyday courage in a young woman coming to terms with a much more complex and baffling world than anything that one not similarly challenged could imagine. Needing to comprehend the disease but realizing the limitations of our clinical explanations; accepting the fact of her diagnosis but resisting its claim on her life; hating phenobarbital but accepting her dependence on it and, courageously, even admitting that she wants more than needs it. Alyssa's poems remind us, as physicians, how the people we are honored to care for must come to terms with problems so much more daunting than we face in our everyday clinical experience, and how much we benefit from their generosity of spirit in sharing their insight with us.

Gerald Novak, MD

SHORT CIRCUIT

AN EPILEPTIC JOURNEY

Alyssa D'Amico

SHIRES 🏛 PRESS

Manchester Center, Vermont

SHIRES ✺ PRESS

4869 Main Street
P.O. Box 2200
Manchester Center, VT 05255
www.northshire.com

Short Circuit
An Epileptic Journey

ISBN: 978-1-60571-386-1

Printed in the United States of America

For my parents, family, friends and all
the people who have helped me through
the years.

Thank you to Michael Geffner and Marvin
Mendlinger from Inspired Word NYC for
giving me the encouragement and
confidence I needed.

Thank you Shelly for all your great ideas.

CONTENTS

That which does not kill us
makes us stronger.

Friedrich Nietzsche

SINGING A SONG

Pheno - combining chemical compounds
Barbital – a barbiturate with white crystalline
powder. Used as a sedative.

Phenobarbital – an addictive, sedative, anti-
depressant, anti-epileptic drug
Overdoses can be fatal

I am medically addicted and
Sometimes want more than needed
On it for 8,401 days of my life
And it ain't over yet

Always above average with the amount of milligrams
Make sure her levels are upper 40's or 50's
No longer able to tell side effects
Because it barely shows
My body and brain depend on it

Wait, I'm feeling nervous today
Don't want an emotional seizure to happen
Should I sneak an extra 16.2 or 64.5 milligrams?
Feeling slightly sedated
Eyes are watery, pupils dilated
It's not noticeable

The fear left
After all it will eventually digest

Do I want a drink?
Only if I'm willing to die
Or skip a dose
Causing a convulsion and controversy

Damn, I'm dizzy
Is it the medication or me?
Give me a seat
Someone pass me a bite to eat
I am shaking like a leaf

Don't continue this fight
Tolerance is going low
Aggressiveness is increasing
It is time to scream!!!
Muscles are getting tight
Let's not continue to fight!

Deeply depressed on and off
Leave me alone!
Clear-headed
Thinking of nothing
Or flashbacks flying through my head
Lying alone to cry away
Less social

Listening to music describing myself
Some of those are so unhappy,
How can that cheer you up?
When will this depression end?
Why did anything happen?
Is there a meaning for me to be alive?
Finally, my pieces are put back together

My memory is perfect
Yet others say no
Medication can affect that so much
Remember there's a learning disability?
No and I will never agree!

Fluctuating fuzzy vision
Everything suddenly looks
Like Van Gogh painted it
Daydreaming? Give me a gold medal
Dreams so vivid
Let's turn it into a fiction story or poem
You want to know what it was about?
Having hallucinations
Don't worry I know that monster isn't real
Let me tell you…
Remind me, did that really happen or
Was it a wish?

Voices heard
Music lines singing in my mind
Are these auras or am I going to overdose?
It can happen either way

Discovering delusions
Stories made up
Acting like a nocturnal animal
Falling asleep four o'clock
More forgetful
Emotions unsteady
No longer sure about fact or fiction
Time to lower it again?
I'm only on the second highest dose
In the hospital I attend

I'm feeling a small withdrawal
Dizziness, and psychiatric
Seizures occurring
A few days in a row
Don't feel any different!
Others claim I am!
"Clearer"
"Quicker"
"More aware"

I don't know what to say
Face the facts, things can be hard to ignore
I'm even afraid to come off
It's been too long
That's why I feel like singing this song
I am medically addicted and
Sometimes want more than needed
Phe-no-bar-bi-tal

STUPIDITY

A virus being shared
No matter how young the kids are
Some parents made them go in anyway
Fevers don't matter
Make the kids suffer
Ignoring how the child isn't feeling well
Not caring how it could be shared
Just to keep their reputation and grades
Running good and high
Perfect attendance! Wow!
Teachers not able to say anything
Principal holding herself back
To not cause trouble
Other parents having concern
Worried and annoyed
It can be dangerous
Help, because some are now sick
Trapped inside at home
Fevers going up
Getting cared about
Hoping that nothing will happen
When will this winter be over?
With how others are acting out of stupidity
Why can't health be understood?
Doctors are out there
To make parents understand
Or are they too ignorant?
And tired of it?

UNKNOWN INFECTION

An unknown viral infection
Low immune system
Temperature going over 104°
Not one doctor was able to
Define the disease
Mother caring for her
Doing everything possible
Until there was a dark night
Continuously calling her
"Come out of the bathroom.
It's time for bed!"
Walked in and saw her body stiff
And head back
Not having a clue on what to do
Tried to wake her up
But there was no response

Rushing to an emergency room
What could possibly be wrong?
Will she wake up?
Is my daughter going to die?
Crying away
Finally, her daughter woke up
A tiny six year old
Short and skinny
Getting a spinal tap over and over
Crying, "Make them stop,
Mommy, make them stop!!!"

A spinal tap being done
Several times in a row
Unfortunately, Mom was held back
From the door of the room
Watching her being held down
By seven nurses
Until it finally worked
But didn't identify what happened at all

Parents and grandparents waiting
To know what was wrong
Seeing seizures happen every half hour
Falling asleep after each
Talking in between
Still somehow smiling
Not sure about what was going on
Phenobarbital put intravenously
No one diagnosing her
Until her father fought for an MRI to be done
Lying down, she was
Slowly moved into a tube
Making all different loud sounds
Listening to the rules
Not to talk or move
She stayed perfectly still
"How are you?"
Her mother asked on and off
"Good," she replied

When over, and slowly moved out
The workers were astonished
She stayed so calm
And walked out standing straight
Not losing any happiness

Then what happened was finally defined
A seizure disorder
Scar tissue was detected
On the left temporal lobe
What is there to do?
Will be found out soon.

MOMMY

Mommy, is a seizure a bad thing?
Does it really make me more stupid?
"Not at all. You are still the same.
Ignore it if you hear that."

Am I gonna die?
Could you sleep with me tonight? I'm scared.
"You know I always do. There is a couch
for both of us."
Yeah, he, he, he.

Mom, could you ever know what will
happen the next day?
"There are usually plans, but sometimes not
everything happens, and
you know what a surprise is."

Why do bad things happen?
Why did I have to get epilepsy?
"There is a reason for everything. You have
to stay strong and never go against yourself."
I love you.
"Now let's get some sleep."

COME BACK

Missing weeks of that winter
The first grade teacher
Had students create get well cards
On construction paper
Multi-colored markers
Small drawings
A few sentences
Saying, "Get better."
"I miss you." "Come back soon."
The principal allowing her to stay
Even though she had to skip day after day
Friends met outside of school
Eventually got to see what was happening to her
When asked by one, "What is a seizure?"
She explained, "It's when the axons shoot neurons in
the wrong directions."
Causing the friend to have a puzzled face
Being seen having one
Learning neurological terms
From hearing them over a lot
Willing to learn
Not cry
But instead asking what that is or,
What does that mean
Carrying on with a high self-esteem

NURSES

When in grammar school I had so many cool nurses
Every time I felt an aura occur
I had to tell the teacher or student near by
If able to walk downstairs
A teacher would ask all 35 students in my class,
"Who wants to be Alyssa's nurse?"
So many friends would raise their hands
I remember Greg the most
Saying to me, "My mom's a nurse. I'm like her."
He was always the cutest to me
When downstairs the secretary would take care of me
Watching the seizure happen
When over, she would decide if I must be picked up
By my parents
Sometimes I really had no choice

Other points of time, I would pass out on the desk
Someone would need to tell the teacher
Or walk out of the classroom to get an adult
Watching me unconscious
Twitching and sucking
Young wondering what was happening
Not sure what to think

When once again waking up
Seeing me in a nervous state of mind
Called postictal
Looking in different directions

11

Asking, "Did I have a seizure?"
Over and over again
"Did I have a seizure?"
Minutes later getting asked, "Are you ok?"
The teacher double-checking that
I was stable enough to stay

WAITING

Once again brought to an emergency room
In Long Island Jewish Hospital
The first attended,
An admission desk on the left
Blue seats connected to the wall
Around a rectangular room
A young girl waiting
Not fully sure
About everything happening around her
Asking Mom, "What's wrong with that person?"
When seeing people unable to walk
Drooling
A skinny elder man with glasses sitting across
Tilting his head to the left
Moving his arms
With a grown woman on the same side
Talking to him
It must have been his daughter
All her mother would say is, "Don't point, that's
not polite. There is just something wrong."
She would sit there waiting for hours
Sometimes until 12am
Other times until 4am
Talking to her mom
Falling asleep on her arm
Her father would go to the desk asking,
"Is she going to be taken in next?"
Finally her name was called
The nurses were dressed all in white

13

With a skirt
Long sleeve shirt
An old-fashioned nurse hat
Only thing, an intern took the blood
It was simple because her veins always showed
But he forgot to connect a tube at the end
And blood went shooting all over the place
Until a nurse pushed him with her whole body
Saying, "GET OUT OF MY WAY!"
Catching it just in time
After taking the needle out
The nurse asked the little girl,
"What Band-Aid do you want?"
She pointed to one with the Power Rangers
Exiting the room through another door
Continuing to wait
Now lying down on a gurney
Sleeping and enjoying her dreams
Finally placed in the Children's Neurology Center
Woken up when brought to a room
For a hep-lock to be placed in her
In case a serious seizure was to occur

Oh NO!! Now it's time for an electroencephalogram
Also know as an EEG
Lying back on the bed
With electrodes being glued to her head
Connected to wires
On the frontal, temporal, occipital lobes
To record the seizures
A needle injecting glue under each

14

Needing to be updated every now and then
She spoke to the EEG technologist
And Mother, as it was put on
A net was put over her head
To keep them in place
Don't touch it! Don't chew gum!
Take all jewelry off!
The wires were plugged into a rectangular box
With a long wire
To keep track of brainwaves
See where the seizures came from
If there were abnormal brain waves
Don't forget two cameras, so if a seizure occurs
It is recorded from every direction
Press the button if you feel or see anything
Yet still able to walk in the room
Her father then went back home
Mother always stayed
To see the doctor the next day
It was a routine that was continually seen

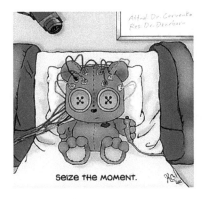

SeIZe THe MOMeNT.

AURA

Prediction of a seizure
Movie scenes flashing through the mind
Making emotions change so quickly
Eyes twitch or stare thinking of it
Slight loss of hearing
Viewing
Drug dealing
Rape
Roger Rabbit cartoons being melted to bits
The Fox and the Hound
Todd needs to find a place to stay
Joy Ride, Rusty Nail destroyed the joy in both boys
Cause of how he is a violent stalker
Who refused to go away
Thinking of past tense pain
Parkside Hospital
Being stuck in an emergency room for hours
Seeing the face of an ex
Trying to escape a mysterious maze
That has pretty dreary coloring
Hearing voices come around saying
What is happening
And what to do
Music lyrics heard out of nowhere
Sights that can only be seen by me
Until everything is over

TINY TEACHER

Third grade the seizures were out of control
Happening almost everyday
Going with Mom to work
Helping to control the children in PS 7
Workers saying, "She's so cute and
looks just like you!"
Is a comment her mother heard at the beginning

Getting a free lunch
Socializing with adults
Some giving her work to do
To help and have fun with a kindergarten class
Passing paper and pens out
Telling them to sit down
Walking with the para in front of the students
Making sure they held hands
"Go to a worker you know, if you feel any aura,"
Her mother said
She never stood alone
Unless delivering something to another classroom

All of a sudden an aura would come
Movies flashing through her mind
She automatically sat down
Going unconscious
With the right eye twitching
Sucking
And right hand shaking
Whoever was around would sit down

Timing it
Taking care of her and,
Trying to call her mother in time
Nervously waking up
Looking around her
Needing some space,
Once fully awake
Spending the rest of the day with Mom
In and out of the school aid office
Where there were three others to talk with
A new person never hurt
One of them would send her to the office
To bring messages
And punch them back in after lunch
The principal had so much respect
Allowing her to be there
After a period of time
Almost all the workers knew her name
Fuhgeddaboudit, one teacher
She was forbidden to go to
Supposedly, she did witchcraft

Today she laughs at that
Not being afraid
Nor was she ever
Yet one para would get paranoid,
"She's a brave little brat,
facing being epileptic."

NOT ENOUGH

Neurosurgery was recommended 1996
Running across a well noted doctor
Making an appointment with him
But a description of scar tissue and seizures
Just wasn't enough
Hearing his response,
"I don't do those simple kinds of brain surgery.
I only do more serious brain surgeries."
Looking back today
Worldwide noted or not
I don't give him one bit of credit
With such a disrespectful remark
Faces can fool you
When the attitude is different inside
Instead acting stubborn
Irresponsible
Bad-mannered
God-like
Five years later
He ironically passed away
After practicing as a neurosurgeon
All his life,
He died because of brain damage
He helped over 2500 people
Except for me
I wonder did he say that remark to other patients too?
It doesn't matter anymore
After all his work is done

AMAZING

An amazing neurosurgeon
Able to help or cure
Epilepsy, injury, cerebral palsy,
And a few other things
Was recommended
For I was a perfect Candidate
Seizures out of control
Dangerous
Happening everyday
Only at the age of eight
The brain not fully grown
Not understanding
What was spoken about
Just simply going along with the show
MRI, MEG, EEG, PET
Left temporal lobe controlling
Math, Speech, Language,
Reading, Cognitive Memory
Why are all those words capital?
Because damage was caused
After all mapping was not done
To see exactly where a seizure comes from
"It is not necessary, not important!"
"Only filing needs to be done."
"Scar tissue is no ordeal."
"She'll be healed!!"
What was said during the appointments?
Is a wonder of my own
Because he ended up being so disappointing

Seizures still out of control
As bad as when I walked in
Just add an LD to me
Learning Disability
Within the cognitive memory
Reading in reverse
Needing to ask how to pronounce words
Getting help for short-term memory
Whenever that name is now heard today
It is annoying and puts me through pain
The only recommendation is not to go to him
Obviously he is of no use!

WORDS

Words running through the mind
Making the head spin
One word is up
The other is down
One full of love
The other is hate
Seeing one on and off in the thin air
Was that missaid?
How many syllables does it have?
Only New Yorkers say it like that?
To say a "th" the tongue touches the top teeth?
It depends on the accent?
What does that mean?
Give a reminder again
How is it pronounced?
That's a double negative?
How is it spelt?
Say it slow
What was the last letter said?
Can you just spell it again?
For a double check
Thanks, pass a dictionary over, let's practice!
Write it continuously?
Say it out loud?
See if it works
Am I able to read now?

Or is the hippocampus moving slow?
Then again, I do not have a hippocampus on that side
Maybe it's medication?
How could that be?
It is not even tellable what it is and isn't from

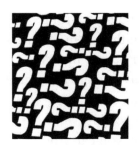

EXTRA TIME

Please give extra time for tests
Or else it may not be finished
Especially for writing
I could move in reverse
Calm down
Don't curse
There is nothing wrong
Just go in that extra room
Made for people like you
Others say you are as normal
As anyone else
A strong person
With how you carry on
But sometimes that can be hard to believe
You never know what will happen next
Go from top grades
To one of the lowest in the class
Feeling like there is no way to move on
Wondering, "Am I gonna get held back?"
"What high school will do?"
"Where can I get to?"

RECOMMENDATIONS

Try a disability public school
I will possibly do better
Parents listened so fast
Chatting with my original friends
On the brand new AOL online
So cool!
Keeping in touch
Still getting together on and off

One day I got so upset
That I ran out of IS 119
Called Joann 718-862-5947
And told her to pick me up
Before they catch up and hit me down to the ground
There was no control
Workers were fools
Just on time
Joann was there with care

SKIPPING

Skipping class
So no one would see her around
Talking to the nurse
Crying about problems
Usually calling her grandparents
To pick her up
Since they lived in the same neighborhood

Out early
At their house
Raising her voice
Ranting and Raving
How she gets mistreated in
The new school
And that there was nothing much to learn
The workers
Had barely any concern for her
They tried to calm her down
But it didn't work

Her parents came
To pick her up
With smiles on their faces
While she looked at them in a state of fury
Making disrespectful remarks
"What are you so happy about?"
Ready to fight about that topic
Then suddenly they said,
"You're going back to OLM!"

She was in a state of shock
Overjoyed
Telling friends
How she was coming back
The next day
Once again walking to the third floor
To Sister Francisca's classroom
When slowly turning the doorknob
The lights went on, out of nowhere
"Surprise!" was screamed out of everyone's mouth
Getting to walk around
And talk early in the morning
Feeling once again happy and welcome

PUT 'EM UP

Keppra is one of the best epileptic medications
But stayed on me for only a number of days
Let's put it this way
Less than a month
My father raised his voice to me
By the door of where we lived
And my reaction was,
Holding my fists like a boxer,
Saying, "Put 'em up! Put 'em up!"
Acting like Oscar De La Hoya
Jumping, maybe I watched
Too many boxing matches
With family
Needed to be calmed down by Mom
Giving her difficulty
Parents looked at each other
Thinking the same
Take her to the hospital
There is something wrong
With how she's acting once again
It must be the medication

CONVERSATION

An adolescent patient
Walking in to see her neurologist
"I would recommend for her to have a second surgery
done. Are there any questions?" the doctor asked
"I would like to ask a question privately"
"Sure." He said and told her parents to get out
She got close, sitting down and said,
"What do you want to do? Crack my head open?"
"Yes! That is what I want to do! Crack heads open to
help children like you. That is what I live for!"
Staring in each other's eyes with anger inside
Only an inch away
Him stamping out
And parents startled
Not knowing what to say

A second operation taking place
Only a bit is being removed
That's not much
Left temporal lobe is not, after all,
The most dangerous kind
60 to 80% chance to help
7% for damage to be done
This is going to be so much fun!
Fear forced inside

Mapping done
Medication being taken off to
Safely see where the removal will be

Waiting for a seizure to happen
Suddenly one occurred
It is now time for the surgery to take place
After a few days
Finally it is done
She was let free
Walking out the hospital door
Until a seizure once again occurs
Unconscious and down
Shaking and sucking
Take her back in
Connect another EEG
Let's see what happened
Falling deeply asleep
Which way did the brain waves move?
A new research to do
Waiting patiently to be let free
And for it to end

DOTS OF BLOOD

Stitches are too simple to take out
Staples are put through the skull
To have the bones grow back together
Not able to wash it with soap
Removed after four days
Twenty-seven in
Pulled out one at a time
Pain every time
"Don't whine! You are strong."
Eyes watering
Still talking
While seeing dots of blood
Finally done
And time to go
It will be fully healed in six to twelve months
Don't worry, some of the hair will grow back
You'll never be fully bald
Touch it as little as possible
Because it could get itchy
If it hurts take an Advil
That can always help
Tylenol can interfere with medication levels
Come back in about three months
So we can do a check up

LOOK AT

When back in school
People and students knew
What she went through
Some asking, "Where was it done?"
Lifting her hair and showing the scar
Some speechless and others
Had responses and comments or asked more
Telling her mom who it was showed to
Almost everyday
Her mother had to explain
How it didn't need to be shared with anybody
And not to answer every question
It's not cool
So don't think it is something to show off
At first she didn't understand
But learned over time how it was wrong
And to stop
Make a part in the center or on the right
So it will not show
A low ponytail is better
Don't make braids in that section
Brush your hair not your head
That may hurt
Especially that it is still fresh
But no matter what remember,
"You will always be the best!"

PERFECT PATIENT

Again another surgical recommendation
From the same doctor at NYU
What could you do?
This is going to be the third time
But is almost fully guaranteed
95 to 98% chance of it working
Why, isn't it worth it?
Seeing some of the most well-known neurologist
For a second opinion
Traveling to Yale for one
Talking on the phone with another on the west coast
Every person saying, "Yes, she is a good candidate
for this. It is definitely going to work."
By 2001
She understood more of what would be done
There was not a fight
This time she went along with it
Still having a small fear
Sometimes going into the hospital
Made her upset
Whether it was for medication, or seizure activity
But let's make this decrease and finally end
Surgery will be the solution
Schedule a date
So she will be prepared
And all tests can be done
To make sure everything that takes place is right
"And done properly concerning me."

FAVORITES

Talking to the nurse practitioner, Alison
As her parents would listen to the surgeon,
They would discuss so many things
Music, cute boys, friends, family, class,
Seizures, nicknames, movies
Some of her favorite games
Eighth grade graduation and prom
So that person knew all her secrets
But was very confidential with it
Keeping a smile on her face
And promised to be there during the surgery

CAUGHT IN A STORM

What a beautiful day! Winters just a comin' and it is beginning to snow. I lay looking up at the flakes falling on me, and around myself was all white. I was even getting buried in it. There was a bar by my feet, flowers all on the left, Alice in Wonderland hiding away from hideous characters yet looking to help. Imagination can run wild in my head. In real life, none of this could be said. All of this is a fiction and lie.

In real life, I was lying in a surgical room. With all white walls, large lights shining down. Feeling tickles of oxygen hit my brain. It was so insane. Seeing slight centimeters of it. Surrounded by six different doctors and a surgeon standing behind. Hearing their voices and what I needed to say in order to keep away from my speech. The flowers were Doctor Bloom, the bar was Doctor Barr, and Alice in Wonderland was Alison, the nurse practitioner that knew my little secrets, promising to be there. After a period of time, I lost myself repeating the alphabet over and over. Alison then jumped out from behind the bushes to help by asking the final questions in order for the surgery to end. For my secrets were finally let out. What might they be?
Here is a list in order for you to see!

Alison: What is your nickname?

Alyssa: IA

Alison: What does IA stand for?

Alyssa: Italian and American

Alison: Who's cute?

Alyssa: Frankie, he's the best!

Alison: Who's better N'Sync or the Backstreet Boys?

Alyssa: N'Sync, they're N'Stink! The Backstreet
Boys are better!

What a giggle we heard out of all the doctors'
mouths. Then again we were the only females in the
room and who can ever know better than us. After the
questions it was time to stop. For the surgeon felt he
was too close to speech and is now done with this
piece. On the way, getting out of the snow, I fell into
a deep sleep while listening to a present from the
surgeon, the song, "The Real Slim Shady."

DID IT WORK?

The answer is no
A complex partial happened
Only thing this time
When she was still in
The surgeon stopped by that night
Discussing it with her mother
Waking her up
"Hi Dr. Lloyd," she said
Smiling with an EEG on her head
He showed how it upset him
She asked questions to fully understand
What happened and why it may not have worked

Basically the whole Hippocampus
Was removed from the left temporal lobe
A fake skull put over the incision
Unseeable and never feel it
Eight baby scars formed
Centimeters long
Like tiny circles
One in the back center of the skull
As Mom always said,
"Don't forget to cover the hole in your head."

MILES

Friends coming to visit me
After the surgery
On the way stopping at FAO Schwarz
Buying this adorable stuffed dog
While trying to figure out what its name should be
Dr. Miles walked in to check up on me
And the response he got was,
"I'm gonna name him Miles. Like you!"
His face turned red, blushing
Yet very happy
A promise was made that
If I ever got a real dog
That would be his name

TIME'S UP

Time's up
And she is finally out
There's no place like home
Take the EEG wires off her head
Such a smelly chemical liquid
Pack those bags up
Get dressed
Here's a hat to cover the glue on your head
Now jump in Dad's car
He's out front
Continuously talking
Then finally home
Walking upstairs
Holding Miles in her arms
Taking the hat off
Having dried glue
Rain from her head to toe
Getting on everything around her
Let's wash her hair
Before it gets all over
Washing it up to eight times in a row
Brushing the knots out
And combing the scalp
To get enough of the glue off
Don't do it over there anymore
Or else she will get a cut
Be most gentle on the left side
Try to do it around, not on top, of the scar
Sitting there for almost an hour

Certain things were so hard in the 90's
The glue didn't change until the early 21st century
Don't worry we got most of it out
More will come off every time
She washes and brushes her hair
And it will eventually be all gone

HORRIBLE HIGH SCHOOL

The first high school attended
The workers were unprofessional
Except for three
Every time a seizure happened in the nurse's office
She was a disrespectful, irresponsible, smart ass
Laughing at, ignoring me
Being looked at by other students and asked,
"What's wrong? Why are you being ignored?"
My shoulders would just go up
With a facial expression
Social fights
Acted like the Wicked Witch of the West
Putting her index finger in front of my eye
Saying, "I see you," for a minute or two
Mom went in to have a discussion
And settle things with her
But that didn't work
The best part is that the nurse
Remembered Mom from high school
But neither her or a friend remembered the nurse
This may have made it worse
Complaints put in
But that did not do much
Even making statements to me
When I was fine
Walking in the hallway
Skipping or changing class

Never got in trouble for anything
Thank Christ the King High School
Only in regard to that

GYM TEST

Hanging out with friends
Sitting on the floor of the gym
Waiting for the teacher to come in
Midterm time
So today is the test
You need to do sit-ups, push-ups
And run a mile
Sit-ups are simple
Make us do more!
Push-ups can be a challenge
But running not sure
It was a steaming hot day
And had to be done outside
After running around the track four times
You were done
Student after student sitting down
Until I was the only one
Asking to stop
Out of breath
Over dizzy
Not sure if I was going to pass out
But she refused for it to end
Unfortunately, the bell didn't ring yet
All of my friends got up and went around
With me and holding me
Making sure I wouldn't fall
Finishing the last round with me
Then giving an applause when done
Saying how great I was

Passing water over
Watching the teacher
Walk away
When ready we walked to the changing room
To get back in our usual uniforms
Ring, Ring, Ring time to learn religion

RACISM AND RELIGION

On the first day in religion class
There were only seven students
When the teacher entered
She said, "You, sit in the back!"
With an attitude tone of voice
Looking at me
I asked, "Why?"
"Go in the back," she replied
African American teacher
Having other students repeat her,
"Get to the back of the room."
"No whites allowed up front."
Until I moved
Somehow listened to rules
After all when it comes to religion
It is important to believe
God is the only one that can understand
Everything

Why listen?
When her voice is unbearable
Why stay?
When being the minority
Why work hard?
When it doesn't count
Why not just walk out?
When no one gets mad
Why give a care?

SCHOOL OF MY DREAMS

I got accepted to the high school of my dreams
Was so excited to start
Located in the city
One of the most fun places to be

The classes are smaller and better
Students I met before time were so much fun
But then things changed
New building, new location
Surrounded by all these spiteful, bitchy people
Who were so well to do
Not willing to accept
The middle class
Living in Queens was not the thing
Acting differently
Polo Sport was so cool

They placed me in the lowest classes
My parents agreed it wasn't the right stage for me
But they refused to change them
Even concerning art and that is a talent inside

Friends?
The only one met who was good
Is a boyfriend that understood
As Kelly Clarkson says,
"I know that I've got issues
but you're pretty messed up too"

No matter what, we accepted each other
And love grew day after day
That will never go away

YOUR FAULT

Seeing you again
Leaves turning red and gold
River water sparkling
Cool air, energy pulsating
People walking, running, laughing

Flowers and plants drying
Brown grass, bare tree limbs
It is fall, and once again I fell

Seeing you again
Memories return
Your promises are like the seasons
Born in the spring, dying in the fall
It's all your fault

It is all because of you
That my brain is once again going insane
Abnormal electrical activity
Neurons are extremely active
Firing off
Making seizures occur
Most happening because of emotions or stress
Over no longer having you
When originally thinking we had another chance
You simply disappear
No longer answering a text

Amount of milligrams going up
Mental side effects developing
From new memories being with
And losing you
I sit and wait for stress to leave
Emotions to be stable
Seizures to decrease
Brain waves more under control
Playing a more proper role
It is all because of you
It's all your fault
All your fault

DRINK

Depressed after having her heart broken
Drinking mudslides midday, at a bar near college
On medications that can cause levels to go off,
A coma or die
Let's hope a seizure doesn't happen

A strange man noticing
That she wasn't walking right
Able to fall, with watery eyes
Not able to talk without a slurry voice
He offered help
Then held her up
Found out about her condition
Walking to Saint Luke's Hospital
Not that much further

Finally when getting there
He described everything possible
And waited for her to get in
Which was really quick
Then wished her good luck
While waiting she wasn't sure what to think of
When asked what was wrong
She slurred, "I take phenobarbital and drank."
They investigated her consciousness
If understanding
"Does the stomach need to be pumped?"
"Should she be admitted?"
"Let's give her some time and see if she gets better."

Lying down for hours
Waiting to know if anything needed to be done
Getting tired of it
Finally a doctor walked in
Deciding that nothing needed to be done
Relax and you can leave in a bit
When time to discharge
She lied about everything
So others would not find out
Different name, phone number, address and ID

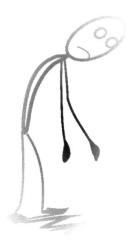

SEIZURE TIME

A seizure
Doesn't please ya
Like a body teaser
Fall to the ground
With no sound
Shaking round and round
People looking down
Thinking what they see
Just let that person be
Don't get too close
This ain't no joke
As a matter of fact, it's no good
Call 911 like you should
Stop having your fun
Try and help!
Or else that person can just melt
And
Have no more life or health

POSTICTAL: THE AFTERMATH

"Was I mean?"
"Do I know everything that is seen?"
"What happened again?"
"I don't remember that."
"You must be kidding?"
Feeling nervous, hyper and barely aware
Now I'm scared!
Moving my head in all different directions
Not sure of what I see or say
"Did I…Did I have…"
"Where did you say?"
"That's where you want me to go?"
"Nooo…"
"Leave me alone!"
"I don't care!"
"It was just a stare."
"No ordeal, let's get real."
"Wait, was I mean?"
"Did I go against the team?"
"Am I a normal human being?"
"I don't know where to be!"
"Not sure, I see…"
"Just bring me home and
not leave me alone, waiting for a room."
Here comes another week of doom

VIMPAT

On Vimpat
Vicious
Irritating
Mental
Poor patients
Abnormal actions
Threatening

A beautiful spring day
Getting ready
For the next course
Just finished making
A perfect power point 2010
Printed it
Then fell backwards
Unable to get up
Still somewhat aware
At 125 pounds
Her father picked her up somehow
She was acting differently
Lying down on the couch
While their puppy Miles was licking her away
Father trying to stop Miles
But she hit him away every time
He immediately called his wife
When home
Mom wasn't even allowed near
911 was called quick
Put into the ambulance

With an oxygen mask on
Because she was not breathing properly
In a detrimental condition
Her father was fighting with the EMT
To bring her to NYU and not Elmhurst Hospital
Which took a while to work
Driving to the city
Only remembering
Being rushed through
The halls of the hospital
And falling asleep
The doctor had to take her off of Vimpat
A medication she was on for a year
AN EEG on as usual
Being told to press the button
If a feeling, a suicidal thought or seizure occur
Keep her in until
She is in good condition
To once again be free
You want a Wii to play?
Having a hep-lock
In her right wrist
She was a lefty for a week and a half
Finally time to leave
After about nine days
Back in college
Everyone that knew her said,
"You look happier."
That was interesting to her
She didn't know how different
It made her act

How it caused such heavy depression
To happen
Secrets and ideas were hidden

But now free from Vimpat

Vicious
Irritating
Mental
Poor patients
Abnormal actions
Threatening

SEX SCENE

Allowed to get up out of bed
For a limited amount of exercise
Let's unplug the EEG
Carry the box in a beautiful blue recyclable bag
Only in the long hallway
"What window do you want to walk to first?"
Asked the nurse
"The right since it is night."
Socializing with the nurse
Walking toward the window
Counting how many workers are still in the building
Across the street
Like playing, *Where's Waldo?*
Who will win finding more?
Are they going to keep score?
"Let's turn around now and
walk to the other window." the nurse said
So they did a 180-degree twist
Walking in the opposite direction
Almost there
Finally looking out the window
Watching the cars drive by
How many bikes were around at that hour?
Then all of a sudden looking in the windows of an
Apartment building across the street
The patient saw such a sex scene
Two people doing it
With the blinds open
The guy on the bottom

Must have been screaming
"Get it in!!"
She then looked at the nurse and said,
"Their having sex!"
The nurse at first didn't notice
Then said, "They are having sex.
Don't they want privacy?"
The patient said, "Does anyone want privacy in that
building? I mean the blinds are always open on
almost every window!"
"True, true, but let's start waking back and stop
watching a live sex show!" The nurse told her
They laughed away
Making fun of those people
Seeing what they had
Time is up and back to the room
"Let's get plugged in and don't forget
you can't get out of bed or go to the bathroom
without pressing the button to tell us."
All the patient said back was,
"Thank you very much!"
Still laughing away about what was seen on that day

MEAN

"Was I mean?" is a line I ask on and off
Especially after an active period
Having a seizure or in the hospital
Getting told it is childish, and how
I once again have a low self-esteem

"Mom, was I mean?"
No, you weren't and need to stop that question!

"Mimi, did I say something mean?"
What are you talkin' about? What did you say
wrong? Not a thing girl!

"Joey, was I mean?"
No, you weren't mean! Say it again and lose our
nickname: Son of a Bitch.

"Professor Tester, I said something bad?"
You asked a question. I don't know what you're
talking about!

"Fay, was I mean?"
No, I will pray to God for this to stop!

"Dr. Harrison, I think I was mean."
You just told me about a seizure!

"Dr. Siddhartha, was I mean?"
No, and we need to raise your self-esteem!

"Judge, did I say something wrong?"
NO, and never ask again! I don't know where you get
that from!

"Michael, was I mean?"
No, I don't know why you think that!

"Madeline, I didn't mean anything."
No worries kiddo
"You're not mad?"
No, why would I be?
"I guess it's a question
I ask after recently having a seizure
Or getting out of a hospital"
No big deal!
Talk to you soon.

After hearing that I learned what is right
To make this end
I am building up my self-esteem again.

"BAD WORD"

Suicide can happen for many different reasons
Disorders, syndromes, frustration
Depression, self-esteem, medication
The levels were off
Serious side effects were showing
At least the last four words
Thinking of that word on and off throughout the year
Researching how to commit it
Tempted to try it twice
But holding back
Seeing the word suicide in the thin air
Holding it in
Asking others what to do
Claiming it was a friend
She wanted to forbid
Writing poems about it
Until one day thinking about life
Giving in to the neurologist
She was seeing while on a medication trial
For the past year
Should it be FDA approved?
How many people did this happen to?
Hysterical crying on the doctor's desk
Letting it off her chest
Patiently waiting for a psychiatrist to come
Being placed in the hospital soon
Slowly, but surely taking it off
Needing to press the button
Whenever the thought came to her head

Once again on an EEG
Then finally free and back to normal
A regular self-esteem, no more depression,
frustration
No longer going the wrong direction
Happy with herself and life
But now phobic of new medications
And coming to the word suicide
It is hard to be said
Socially acting like a child
Saying, "the bad word," instead
Now on a different medication
Barely any side effects
Acting and thinking like no one else, but herself

HARD TO ESCAPE

It is hard to escape
When feeling in outer space
How will life be?
What is wrong with me?
I am blinded and cannot see
Fear can sometimes be near
At this point, it is all up to you for what to do
Medication can be noticed
Side effects can show
How many fingers do I see?
You put up one, but I see three
Fuzzy vision
Viewing double
Another delusion
Making up stories
Seizures out of control
Not having a say
Make that headache go away!
Suffering everyday
But don't give up today
A cure is waiting to be found
Doctors searching all around
To figure out what to do
Hospitals can make you feel alone
When in real life
Others are there that do care
Everyone waiting for epilepsy to go and stay away
When feeling in outer space
It is hard to escape

CONTROL LOST

Neurons overactive
Moving in all different directions
Seizure after seizure
Memory lost
Waking up either in a hospital or on the floor
Barely able to walk out the door
Someone needs to be with you
No matter where you go
Whether it's a friend or family
Medication increasing
Causing you to get down in the dumps
Side effects increasing
Not helping a bit
Just sit there and wait
For things to get straight

ALONE

Drop to the ground
With no sound
Surrounded by darkness
Not a person around
To help with these twitches and turns
Times running fast
You never know how long a seizure could last
Hours are too long
Someone come before life is gone
Sent to the emergency room
With people all around
Barely able to understand a word or sound
Going into a deep sleep
Woken up alone in bed
Wondering what happened
Until noticing the hair became ultra-long
In all different colors: red, blue, green, yellow
These wires run tests
To help find which treatment is the best
How long will it take?
No one knows
An EEG can last hours, days or weeks
But try and remember to have no fright
And that everything will be all right
Believe in yourself
Don't lose faith
Something will be found one day
Then everything will be okay

TERROR

In an ambulance
After having a complex partial seizure in New York
People making a mountain out of a molehill
Overly postictal
Full of fear
Wondering why'd this happen?
Where are these people coming from?
Are they going to hurt me?
"Let me free!!!"
"Stop touching me!!!"
Getting more nervous every time a hand touched
"What happened again?"
Repeating, "DID I HAVE A SEIZURE? DID I
HAVE A SEIZURE?"
Squiggling over and over
Hand cuffed to the gurney
No friend or family near
To clam me down
Driven to a hospital
Waiting alone
In an emergency room
Getting looked at by others
What do they think?
Seeing so many more serious cases
With oxygen masks
Wires on the heart
Weird looking objects
That I don't even know what they are
Well, I'm here again

Is all I can say
When still aware
Because I am so used to the atmosphere,
Sights and treatments
How long it can take for a worker to come over
Can even describe some locations
Off the top of my mind
When will a doctor show up?
So I can get out
Anxiety
Getting exhausted
Falling asleep
Not making a peep
Until finally woken
After hours went past
By a doctor checking up
Asking tons of questions,
"Why are you here?"
"Is there a disease or disorder?'
"What kind of seizures do you have?"
"Who is your doctor?"
"Are you on medication?"
"If so, which ones?"
"What is your insurance?"
"Where do you live?"
"Let's check the blood pressure."
"Temperature is a little low, 95.2"
Now it's time to take blood
"Wait, where are the veins?"
I got stabbed by needles one too many times
Since a kid

So now they're hidden
Still they try and get it in
Sitting up straight
Holding the arm still
"Think one was found."
"Wait, it didn't work."
"Show me the other arm."
"Make a fist. Hold it tight."
Touch, touch
It is time to try again
"Missed it."
Let's move the needle to the left
Now to the right
Undo the wrist now
"Finally got one done."
"Good, now let me out!!!"
It is time to discharged
I waited one too many hours

UP AND DOWN

Did the levels go up?
Or head down?
Is it causing depression?
Making the person
Not fully aware of what is going on
Feeling like all that is done wrong
Randomly falling asleep
Turning dreams into real life
Will that hurt?
Wondering why certain things had to happen
Could life change and get better or is that unreal?
Hallucinations standing there
Getting unsure about the real world
Forgetting what was about to be said
Spelling left the person's head
How did that happen?
Tongue twisted
Staring off
Feeling bare
Colors showing up in the air
And like nothing is fair
Or levels going down
Making a seizure happen everyday
The person feels that there is no more to say
Being in and out of the hospital
Admitting knows the person
The name rolls off their tongue
Not knowing what to do
Raise this, lower that, put another on, take that off

How about a diet?
Too hard to keep?
Is it time for surgery?
Life, what is there to do?
Getting interference while at work
Seeing fuzzy
Gaining weight
Losing weight
Not thinking straight
Wishes wanted
Will they eventually come true?
There is help for the person
Having seizure after seizure
Something needs to be figured out
It is time to check the levels
Did they go up?
Or head down?

A DECADE

I'm seeing you for more than a decade
And there are still seizures
So a few things can be tried
But let's not jump to an implant
A new medication came out
But before that you need to get your eyesight checked
Because irreversible blindness is one side effect

Going to a neuro-ophthalmologist
Getting tests done
Finding out I am not qualified
Some peripheral vision was lost

Let's then try the ketogenic diet
That was too hard
Lamictal raised
Causing a loss of balance
In the hospital to lower it
Lamictal level goes down ↓
Phenobarbital level goes up ↑
Needs to be adjusted again
Feeling like the seizures never decreased

A final seizure happening
In the emergency room
Acting different
Thanking the quartz bracelet
Claiming it made her strong enough to live
Waiting, staring off in a different dimension

Falling asleep on and off
Eyes half closed

Needing to get a CAT scan
And something else was done
Forgot what
Then brought up to the room
Nurses trying to get an IV in
Squiggling and refusing
Acting like a child
Then a seizure happened
Sitting, she went backwards
Darn, there was no EEG on
The epileptologist next morning made a decision
Of what would be done
Time to see the surgeon about an implant
Given all details

VOICE IS GETTING HOARSE

With the Vagus Nerve Stimulator
Voice is getting hoarse
On and off
It could be annoying
Surgically placed below the skin of the upper chest
An electrode is attached
To the vagus nerve
In the neck
Feeling as if it is on top of that part
Stimulating every one minute
24/7
Least amount of time
For it to be set on
Randomly coughing
Eyes watering
Overly itchy throat
Losing the voice
Barely able to talk
Or feel pain on the throat
Afraid to talk
Wait patiently for it to go away
Texting is ok
A magnet needs to be worn
Connecting onto metal objects, desk, and walls
Needing to pull it off
Friends find that amusing
It is fun to play with
Making spoons move around in circles
At points of time it feels like a toy

And I think of it as body art
Even though seizures can still start
They are less often and less severe
Most of the time staying aware
But no matter what
It is a scare
They are stopped or only seconds long
By swiping the magnet to the chest
Whenever it is needed to be used
Stimulation traveling
Voice going monotone for about a minute
It may look strange and be misunderstood
Yet worth making the voice hoarse on and off
Don't talk
Wait until it's back to normal some say
But it really doesn't matter
Some asking if my throat was slit
"Where did you get that from?"
"At what age did you get it?"
Interviewers asking questions
It could be annoying
Yet controlling and helpful
On and off the voice getting hoarse
Having a Vagus Nerve Stimulator

FUNKY FRIDAY

An extra 64.5 milligrams was needed
Emotionally
To be in my own little world
In a mad mood or under stress
I can make my mind clear magically
Only with a little extra help

Now I'm upset
Feel under threat
Not sure how I am set
At an event
Unable to understand what a person said,
"Need a dollar?
Here's one.
Wait I have two!"
Taking them out
Stopped by a friend,
"She did not say that
and wasn't talking to you."
Reminding me
I was supposed to go to the vending machine
To buy a healthy drink
Gatorade is good enough
"Am I doing the right thing?"
Double check
I feel desperate
Not even sure if I will be able to perform poetry
Feeling sedated and stoned
Slightly off

Not fully aware
Less emotional
Sometimes no facial expressions
Eyes half way closed
For a period of time

Remind me what I said
Is it a care?
All I can say is, it will eventually digest
Getting quiet
Falling asleep leaning against a wall
Getting looked at every now and then
Told to sit and obey
In this condition a person can get me to do anything

Having conversations and laughing in between
Waiting for my turn to go on
Performing *Singing a Song*
Seeing facial expressions
And that night was done

The next morning
Thanking God I am still alive
While flashing back
Trying to remember as much as possible
Feeling upset with no one other than myself
Since it was all my fault
Being unaware on and off all night
Never do things without a person saying
It is all right

EPILEPSY

Epilepsy is a part of me
You can take it or leave it
Because it may not go away
As a matter of fact
It may be here to stay
Am I ok? Yes I am!
Standing up straight
Facing the reality of life
Accepting every part, and possibility for it
Continuing to carry on
Have fun, enjoy myself, do favorite things
Try to make sure there is a smile on my face
But emotions fluctuate
Not every day is perfect
Life is like a ride going up and down
Researching the condition reminding myself
What the chemistry is
When a seizure happens
Stay strong
There is nothing wrong
Back to normal
Whatever that means
Let me continue with what I am going to do
Epilepsy is a part of me
Which makes me unique
In a different way
Keep my head up
And never give up

Cause winners never quit
Quitters never win
And I chose to be a winner

DIFFERENT GIRL

I am a different girl
From a different world
A different race
With a different face
From another dimension
I am dealing with a different case
I am an unknown species
Unique in many ways
Have an imagination that runs wild
Am able to fly
Because dreams are coming true
I glow in the dark
I am filled with ultimate powers
And have a real heart
Don't have much to say or do
Some people of the world are prejudice against me
Because they don't understand what they see
I am a different girl
From a different world

ACCEPTANCE

What is there really different to see?
About anyone, including me
We are all just the same
Some who have epilepsy are or were in fame
All people are exclusive in their own way
And there is nothing more to say

GLOSSARY

Aura: A warning before a seizure either occurring alone or before a complex partial or generalized seizure. Also, a warning before a migraine headache.

Axon: The part of the nerve cell (neuron) that communicates with other cells, similar to a telephone wire.

Blood drug level: The concentration, or amount of circulating drug in the blood stream measured in micrograms or nanograms per milliliter.

EEG Electroencephalogram: A diagnostic test of brain electrical activity; helpful in diagnosing epilepsy.

Hippocampus: A small organ located in the brain's medial temporal lobe and is an important part of the region that regulates emotions. It is associated mainly with memory, in particular long-term memory.

Levels: see blood drug level

Neuron: A specialized cell transmitting nerve impulse; a nerve cell.

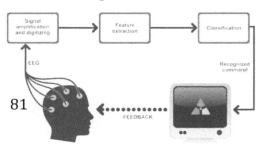

Postictal: Referring to the period immediately after a seizure; the altered state of consciousness after a seizure, lasting between 5 to 30 minutes, and may be characterized by drowsiness, confusion, hypertension or headache.

Seizure: A sudden, excessive discharge of nervous-system electrical activity that usually causes a change of behavior and abnormal electrical discharge in the brain.

Temporal lobe: Located behind your ears and extending to both sides of the brain. It is involved in vision, memory, sensory input, language, emotion and comprehension.

Vagus nerve: The longest of 12 cranial nerves, extending from the brainstem to the abdomen; forming part of the involuntary nervous system commanding unconscious body procedures, such as keeping heart rate constant and controlling food digestion.

Vagus Nerve Stimulator (VNS): A pacemaker-like device, implanted in the upper chest, which stimulates a nerve in the left neck; the VNS sends mild pulses to the vagus nerve at regular intervals throughout the day to try to stop or reduce seizure activity.

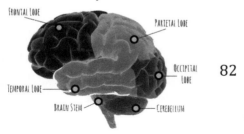

82

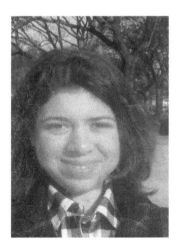

ABOUT THE AUTHOR

Alyssa D'Amico was born and raised in Queens, New York City. At the age of 6, she was diagnosed with epilepsy and started writing poetry soon after. Her work has been published by Albany Poets, Inc. in Up the River, New York University F.A.C.E.S., the National Epilepsy Foundation, and the Epilepsy Foundation of Northeastern New York. She has been a featured poet at the Queens NYC Lit Festival with Inspired Word in 2016 and 2017.

Alyssa's goal is to help people with neurological disorders, including epilepsy, to believe in themselves. She would also like to make people who are not familiar with epilepsy more aware.

CPSIA information can be obtained
at www.ICGtesting.com
Printed in the USA
LVHW01s1941220118
563534LV00015B/1461/P

9 781605 713861